# Introdu

Date of Birth: _____

Gestational Age: _____

Time: _____

Weight: _____

Length: _____

Hospital(s): _____

_____

Delivery Room Doctor(s): _____

_____

_____

Delivery Room Nurse(s): _____

_____

_____

# How to use this Journal

This journal was created as a means of keeping all your baby's information organized in one place and was inspired by a family member's time in NICU with preemie twins. There is no right or wrong way to record your journey, because just as every baby is different, so too will every NICU experience be different.

You can start this journal at anytime, just write the number of the day on the first daily page in the Heart provided. For example if you start this journal on NICU day number 3 then you would write a "3" in the Heart of the first daily page.

If this is your first time in NICU it can be overwhelming. Use this journal as a means to help you remember the important details about your child's care. It can be very useful to write down questions as you think of them so you will not forget them when you have the chance to speak to a doctor or nurse. Do not be afraid to ask the nurses any questions you have or to explain anything you do not understand, especially terminology that is unfamiliar to you.

There are 8 weeks worth of pages (some stays will require another journal and some will not use this one in its entirety). At the end of each week there are "check-in" and "journal pages" for you to reflect on the week and record your thoughts and feelings and any milestones reached. There is also a place each week for a photo or you can use that space to draw, sketch or doodle. The photo space could also be used to track anything that is not included on the daily pages.

# Thoughts About Peanut

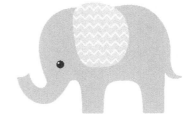

**MY PARENTS ARE GREATFUL FOR:**

**MY PARENTS HOPE THAT I WILL GROW UP TO BE:**

**MY NAME WAS CHOSEN BECAUSE:**

# Visitors

| NAME | DATE |
|------|------|
| | |
| | |
| | |
| | |
| | |
| | |
| | |
| | |
| | |
| | |
| | |
| | |
| | |
| | |

# Goals for...

DATE:

DATE:

DATE:

DATE:

DATE:

DATE:

Date: _____

Gestational Age: _____

NICU Day #

## What We Did Today

Feeding   Phone Call   Video Call

Touch   Diaper   Hold

Skin to Skin   Check Temp   Bath

Visitors   Photos   Rocking Chair

Sing   Read   Massage

Today's Positives   Today's Challenges

Questions To Ask & Notes:

## Today's Doctors ♡

## Today's Nurses ♡

## Equipment & Settings:

## Vital Signs ♡

## Medications & Labs ♡

## Feedings & Procedures:

Date: _____

Gestational Age: _____

NICU Day #

## What We Did Today

Feeding          Phone Call          Video Call

Touch            Diaper              Hold

Skin to Skin     Check Temp          Bath

Visitors         Photos              Rocking Chair

Sing             Read                Massage

Today's Positives ♡        Today's Challenges

Questions To Ask & Notes:

Today's Doctors ♡    Today's Nurses ♡

Equipment & Settings:

Vital Signs ♡    Medications & Labs ♡

Feedings & Procedures:

Date: _____

Gestational Age: _____

**NICU Day #**

## What We Did Today

| | | |
|---|---|---|
| ☐ Feeding | ☐ Phone Call | ☐ Video Call |
| ☐ Touch | ☐ Diaper | ☐ Hold |
| ☐ Skin to Skin | ☐ Check Temp | ☐ Bath |
| ☐ Visitors | ☐ Photos | ☐ Rocking Chair |
| ☐ Sing | ☐ Read | ☐ Massage |
| ☐ | ☐ | ☐ |

### Today's Positives ♡

### Today's Challenges

### Questions To Ask & Notes:

Today's Doctors ♡

Today's Nurses ♡

Equipment & Settings:

Vital Signs ♡

Medications & Labs ♡

Feedings & Procedures:

Date: _____

Gestational Age: _____

NICU Day #

## What We Did Today

Feeding          Phone Call          Video Call

Touch            Diaper              Hold

Skin to Skin     Check Temp          Bath

Visitors         Photos              Rocking Chair

Sing             Read                Massage

Today's Positives ♡          Today's Challenges

Questions To Ask & Notes:

## Today's Doctors ♡

## Today's Nurses ♡

## Equipment & Settings:

## Vital Signs ♡

## Medications & Labs ♡

## Feedings & Procedures:

Date: _____

NICU Day #

Gestational Age: _____

## What We Did Today

| | | |
|---|---|---|
| Feeding | Phone Call | Video Call |
| Touch | Diaper | Hold |
| Skin to Skin | Check Temp | Bath |
| Visitors | Photos | Rocking Chair |
| Sing | Read | Massage |
| | | |

Today's Positives ♡

Today's Challenges

Questions To Ask & Notes:

## Today's Doctors ♡

## Today's Nurses ♡

## Equipment & Settings:

## Vital Signs ♡

## Medications & Labs ♡

## Feedings & Procedures:

Date: _____

Gestational Age: _____

NICU Day #

## What We Did Today

- Feeding
- Phone Call
- Video Call
- Touch
- Diaper
- Hold
- Skin to Skin
- Check Temp
- Bath
- Visitors
- Photos
- Rocking Chair
- Sing
- Read
- Massage

### Today's Positives ♡

### Today's Challenges

### Questions To Ask & Notes:

## Today's Doctors ♡

## Today's Nurses ♡

## Equipment & Settings:

## Vital Signs ♡

## Medications & Labs ♡

## Feedings & Procedures:

Date: _____

NICU Day #

Gestational Age: _____

## What We Did Today

Feeding      Phone Call      Video Call

Touch      Diaper      Hold

Skin to Skin      Check Temp      Bath

Visitors      Photos      Rocking Chair

Sing      Read      Massage

Today's Positives ♡ | Today's Challenges

Questions To Ask & Notes:

## Today's Doctors ♡

## Today's Nurses ♡

## Equipment & Settings:

## Vital Signs ♡

## Medications & Labs ♡

## Feedings & Procedures:

# Weekly Check-In

## NEGATIVE THOUGHTS ONLY HAVE THE POWER I ALLOW THEM

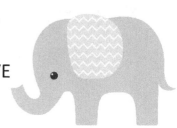

**MILESTONES:**

**UPS & DOWNS:**

**BABY'S LIKES & DISLIKES:**

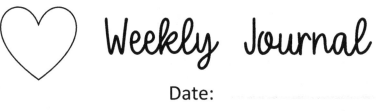

# Weekly Journal

Date:

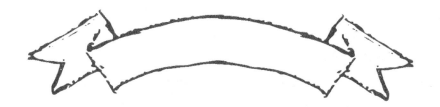

Date: _____

Gestational Age: _____

NICU Day #

## What We Did Today

- Feeding
- Phone Call
- Video Call
- Touch
- Diaper
- Hold
- Skin to Skin
- Check Temp
- Bath
- Visitors
- Photos
- Rocking Chair
- Sing
- Read
- Massage

Today's Positives ♡

Today's Challenges

Questions To Ask & Notes:

## Today's Doctors ♡

## Today's Nurses ♡

## Equipment & Settings:

## Vital Signs ♡

## Medications & Labs ♡

## Feedings & Procedures:

Date: _____

NICU Day #

Gestational Age: _____

## What We Did Today

- Feeding
- Phone Call
- Video Call
- Touch
- Diaper
- Hold
- Skin to Skin
- Check Temp
- Bath
- Visitors
- Photos
- Rocking Chair
- Sing
- Read
- Massage

Today's Positives ♡ | Today's Challenges

Questions To Ask & Notes:

## Today's Doctors ♡

## Today's Nurses ♡

## Equipment & Settings:

## Vital Signs ♡

## Medications & Labs ♡

## Feedings & Procedures:

Date: _____

Gestational Age: _____

NICU Day #

## What We Did Today

Feeding        Phone Call        Video Call

Touch          Diaper            Hold

Skin to Skin   Check Temp        Bath

Visitors       Photos            Rocking Chair

Sing           Read              Massage

---

Today's Positives  ♡        Today's Challenges

Questions To Ask & Notes:

Today's Doctors ♡

Today's Nurses ♡

Equipment & Settings:

Vital Signs ♡

Medications & Labs ♡

Feedings & Procedures:

Date: _____

Gestational Age: _____

NICU Day #

## What We Did Today

- Feeding
- Phone Call
- Video Call
- Touch
- Diaper
- Hold
- Skin to Skin
- Check Temp
- Bath
- Visitors
- Photos
- Rocking Chair
- Sing
- Read
- Massage

Today's Positives ♡

Today's Challenges

Questions To Ask & Notes:

## Today's Doctors ♡

## Today's Nurses ♡

## Equipment & Settings:

## Vital Signs ♡

## Medications & Labs ♡

## Feedings & Procedures:

Date: _____

NICU Day #

Gestational Age: _____

## What We Did Today

Feeding        Phone Call        Video Call

Touch        Diaper        Hold

Skin to Skin        Check Temp        Bath

Visitors        Photos        Rocking Chair

Sing        Read        Massage

Today's Positives ♡

Today's Challenges

Questions To Ask & Notes:

## Today's Doctors ♡

## Today's Nurses ♡

## Equipment & Settings:

## Vital Signs ♡

## Medications & Labs ♡

## Feedings & Procedures:

Date: _____

Gestational Age: _____

NICU Day #

## What We Did Today

- Feeding
- Phone Call
- Video Call
- Touch
- Diaper
- Hold
- Skin to Skin
- Check Temp
- Bath
- Visitors
- Photos
- Rocking Chair
- Sing
- Read
- Massage

Today's Positives ♡

Today's Challenges

Questions To Ask & Notes:

Today's Doctors ♡

Today's Nurses ♡

Equipment & Settings:

Vital Signs ♡

Medications & Labs ♡

Feedings & Procedures:

Date: _____

NICU Day #

Gestational Age: _____

## What We Did Today

- Feeding
- Phone Call
- Video Call
- Touch
- Diaper
- Hold
- Skin to Skin
- Check Temp
- Bath
- Visitors
- Photos
- Rocking Chair
- Sing
- Read
- Massage

Today's Positives ♡

Today's Challenges

Questions To Ask & Notes:

Today's Doctors ♡

Today's Nurses ♡

Equipment & Settings:

Vital Signs ♡

Medications & labs ♡

Feedings & Procedures:

# Weekly Check-In

## DIFFICULT TIMES ARE PART OF MY JOURNEY AND ALLOW ME TO APPRECIATE THE GOOD

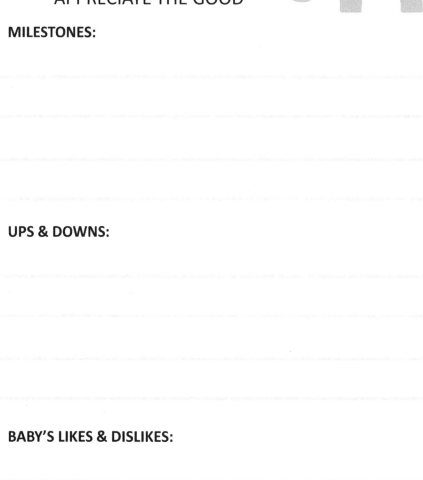

**MILESTONES:**

**UPS & DOWNS:**

**BABY'S LIKES & DISLIKES:**

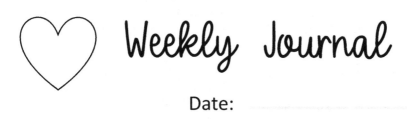

# Weekly Journal

Date:

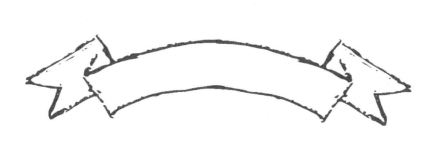

Date: _____

NICU Day #

Gestational Age: _____

## What We Did Today

- [ ] Feeding
- [ ] Phone Call
- [ ] Video Call
- [ ] Touch
- [ ] Diaper
- [ ] Hold
- [ ] Skin to Skin
- [ ] Check Temp
- [ ] Bath
- [ ] Visitors
- [ ] Photos
- [ ] Rocking Chair
- [ ] Sing
- [ ] Read
- [ ] Massage
- [ ] 
- [ ] 
- [ ] 

### Today's Positives ♡

### Today's Challenges

### Questions To Ask & Notes:

Today's Doctors ♡

Today's Nurses ♡

Equipment & Settings:

Vital Signs ♡

Medications & Labs ♡

Feedings & Procedures:

Date: _____

Gestational Age: _____

NICU Day #

## What We Did Today

Feeding     Phone Call     Video Call

Touch     Diaper     Hold

Skin to Skin     Check Temp     Bath

Visitors     Photos     Rocking Chair

Sing     Read     Massage

Today's Positives ♡ | Today's Challenges

Questions To Ask & Notes:

## Today's Doctors ♡

## Today's Nurses ♡

## Equipment & Settings:

## Vital Signs ♡

## Medications & Labs ♡

## Feedings & Procedures:

Date: _____

NICU Day #

Gestational Age: _____

## What We Did Today

- Feeding
- Touch
- Skin to Skin
- Visitors
- Sing

- Phone Call
- Diaper
- Check Temp
- Photos
- Read

- Video Call
- Hold
- Bath
- Rocking Chair
- Massage

---

Today's Positives ♡

Today's Challenges

Questions To Ask & Notes:

## Today's Doctors ♡

## Today's Nurses ♡

## Equipment & Settings:

## Vital Signs ♡

## Medications & Labs ♡

## Feedings & Procedures:

Date: _____

Gestational Age: _____

NICU Day #

## What We Did Today

- Feeding
- Phone Call
- Video Call
- Touch
- Diaper
- Hold
- Skin to Skin
- Check Temp
- Bath
- Visitors
- Photos
- Rocking Chair
- Sing
- Read
- Massage

Today's Positives ♡ | Today's Challenges

Questions To Ask & Notes:

## Today's Doctors ♡

## Today's Nurses ♡

## Equipment & Settings:

## Vital Signs ♡

## Medications & Labs ♡

## Feedings & Procedures:

Date: _____

Gestational Age: _____

### What We Did Today

NICU Day #

- [ ] Feeding
- [ ] Phone Call
- [ ] Video Call
- [ ] Touch
- [ ] Diaper
- [ ] Hold
- [ ] Skin to Skin
- [ ] Check Temp
- [ ] Bath
- [ ] Visitors
- [ ] Photos
- [ ] Rocking Chair
- [ ] Sing
- [ ] Read
- [ ] Massage
- [ ]
- [ ]
- [ ]

**Today's Positives** ♡

**Today's Challenges**

**Questions To Ask & Notes:**

Today's Doctors ♡    Today's Nurses ♡

Equipment & Settings:

Vital Signs ♡    Medications & Labs ♡

Feedings & Procedures:

Date: _____

NICU Day #

Gestational Age: _____

## What We Did Today

- [ ] Feeding
- [ ] Phone Call
- [ ] Video Call
- [ ] Touch
- [ ] Diaper
- [ ] Hold
- [ ] Skin to Skin
- [ ] Check Temp
- [ ] Bath
- [ ] Visitors
- [ ] Photos
- [ ] Rocking Chair
- [ ] Sing
- [ ] Read
- [ ] Massage
- [ ] 
- [ ] 
- [ ] 

### Today's Positives ♡

### Today's Challenges

### Questions To Ask & Notes:

## Today's Doctors ♡

## Today's Nurses ♡

## Equipment & Settings:

## Vital Signs ♡

## Medications & Labs ♡

## Feedings & Procedures:

Date: _____

NICU Day #

Gestational Age: _____

## What We Did Today

Feeding     Phone Call     Video Call

Touch     Diaper     Hold

Skin to Skin     Check Temp     Bath

Visitors     Photos     Rocking Chair

Sing     Read     Massage

Today's Positives ♡     Today's Challenges

Questions To Ask & Notes:

Today's Doctors ♡

Today's Nurses ♡

Equipment & Settings:

Vital Signs ♡

Medications & Labs ♡

Feedings & Procedures:

# Weekly Check-In

NO AMOUNT OF GUILT CAN CHANGE
THE PAST, AND NO AMOUNT OF
WORRY CAN CHANGE THE FUTURE

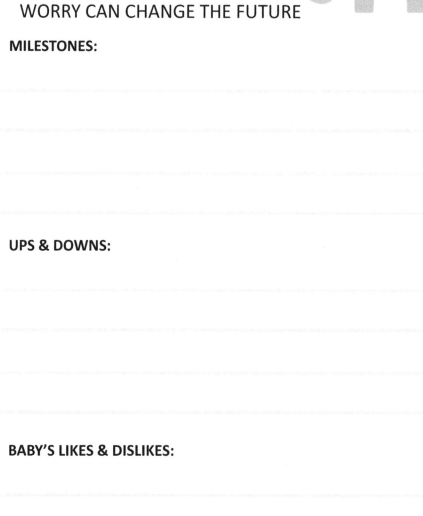

**MILESTONES:**

**UPS & DOWNS:**

**BABY'S LIKES & DISLIKES:**

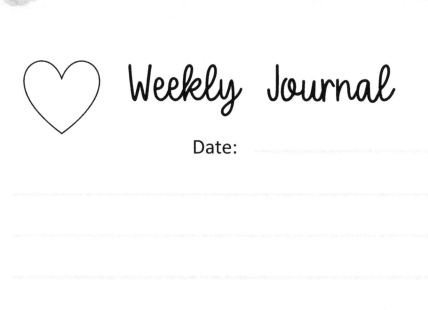

# Weekly Journal

Date: _____

_____

_____

_____

_____

_____

_____

_____

_____

_____

_____

_____

_____

_____

_____

_____

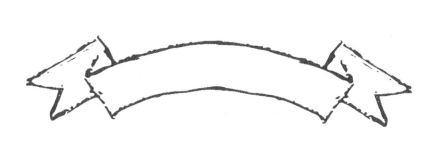

Date: _____

NICU Day #

Gestational Age: _____

## What We Did Today

Feeding     Phone Call     Video Call

Touch     Diaper     Hold

Skin to Skin     Check Temp     Bath

Visitors     Photos     Rocking Chair

Sing     Read     Massage

Today's Positives ♡     Today's Challenges

Questions To Ask & Notes:

## Today's Doctors ♡

## Today's Nurses ♡

## Equipment & Settings:

## Vital Signs ♡

## Medications & Labs ♡

## Feedings & Procedures:

Date: _____

Gestational Age: _____

NICU Day #

## What We Did Today

- ☐ Feeding
- ☐ Phone Call
- ☐ Video Call
- ☐ Touch
- ☐ Diaper
- ☐ Hold
- ☐ Skin to Skin
- ☐ Check Temp
- ☐ Bath
- ☐ Visitors
- ☐ Photos
- ☐ Rocking Chair
- ☐ Sing
- ☐ Read
- ☐ Massage
- ☐
- ☐

Today's Positives ♡

Today's Challenges

Questions To Ask & Notes:

Today's Doctors ♡

Today's Nurses ♡

Equipment & Settings:

Vital Signs ♡

Medications & Labs ♡

Feedings & Procedures:

Date: _____

Gestational Age: _____

**NICU Day #**

## What We Did Today

- Feeding
- Phone Call
- Video Call
- Touch
- Diaper
- Hold
- Skin to Skin
- Check Temp
- Bath
- Visitors
- Photos
- Rocking Chair
- Sing
- Read
- Massage

Today's Positives ♡

Today's Challenges

Questions To Ask & Notes:

## Today's Doctors ♡

## Today's Nurses ♡

## Equipment & Settings:

## Vital Signs ♡

## Medications & Labs ♡

## Feedings & Procedures:

Date: _____

**NICU Day #**

Gestational Age: _____

## What We Did Today

- Feeding
- Phone Call
- Video Call
- Touch
- Diaper
- Hold
- Skin to Skin
- Check Temp
- Bath
- Visitors
- Photos
- Rocking Chair
- Sing
- Read
- Massage

Today's Positives

Today's Challenges

Questions To Ask & Notes:

## Today's Doctors ♡

## Today's Nurses ♡

## Equipment & Settings:

## Vital Signs ♡

## Medications & Labs ♡

## Feedings & Procedures:

Date: _____

NICU Day #

Gestational Age: _____

## What We Did Today

Feeding          Phone Call          Video Call

Touch            Diaper              Hold

Skin to Skin     Check Temp          Bath

Visitors         Photos              Rocking Chair

Sing             Read                Massage

Today's Positives ♡          Today's Challenges

Questions To Ask & Notes:

Today's Doctors ♡

Today's Nurses ♡

Equipment & Settings:

Vital Signs ♡

Medications & labs ♡

Feedings & Procedures:

Date: _____

Gestational Age: _____

NICU Day #

## What We Did Today

- Feeding
- Touch
- Skin to Skin
- Visitors
- Sing

- Phone Call
- Diaper
- Check Temp
- Photos
- Read

- Video Call
- Hold
- Bath
- Rocking Chair
- Massage

Today's Positives ♡

Today's Challenges

Questions To Ask & Notes:

## Today's Doctors ♡

## Today's Nurses ♡

## Equipment & Settings:

## Vital Signs ♡

## Medications & Labs ♡

## Feedings & Procedures:

Date: _____

Gestational Age: _____

NICU Day #

## What We Did Today

| | | |
|---|---|---|
| Feeding | Phone Call | Video Call |
| Touch | Diaper | Hold |
| Skin to Skin | Check Temp | Bath |
| Visitors | Photos | Rocking Chair |
| Sing | Read | Massage |
| | | |

### Today's Positives ♡

### Today's Challenges

### Questions To Ask & Notes:

## Today's Doctors ♡

## Today's Nurses ♡

## Equipment & Settings:

## Vital Signs ♡

## Medications & Labs ♡

## Feedings & Procedures:

# Weekly Check-In

## I AM IN CHARGE OF HOW I FEEL
## AND TODAY I AM
## CHOOSING HAPPINESS

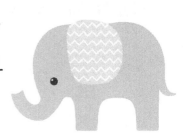

**MILESTONES:**

**UPS & DOWNS:**

**BABY'S LIKES & DISLIKES:**

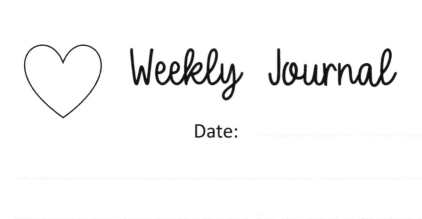

# Weekly Journal

Date:

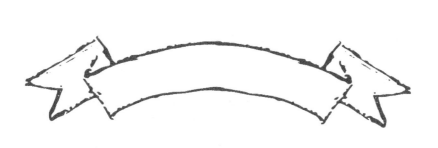

Date: _____

Gestational Age: _____

NICU Day #

## What We Did Today

Feeding          Phone Call          Video Call

Touch            Diaper              Hold

Skin to Skin     Check Temp          Bath

Visitors         Photos             Rocking Chair

Sing             Read               Massage

---

### Today's Positives ♡

### Today's Challenges

### Questions To Ask & Notes:

## Today's Doctors ♡

## Today's Nurses ♡

## Equipment & Settings:

## Vital Signs ♡

## Medications & Labs ♡

## Feedings & Procedures:

Date: _____

Gestational Age: _____

NICU Day #

## What We Did Today

Feeding          Phone Call          Video Call

Touch            Diaper              Hold

Skin to Skin     Check Temp          Bath

Visitors         Photos              Rocking Chair

Sing             Read                Massage

Today's Positives ♡ | Today's Challenges

Questions To Ask & Notes:

Today's Doctors ♡

Today's Nurses ♡

Equipment & Settings:

Vital Signs ♡

Medications & Labs ♡

Feedings & Procedures:

Date: _____

NICU Day #

Gestational Age: _____

## What We Did Today

☐ Feeding      ☐ Phone Call      ☐ Video Call

☐ Touch        ☐ Diaper          ☐ Hold

☐ Skin to Skin ☐ Check Temp      ☐ Bath

☐ Visitors     ☐ Photos          ☐ Rocking Chair

☐ Sing         ☐ Read            ☐ Massage

☐              ☐                 ☐

### Today's Positives ♡

_____

_____

_____

_____

### Today's Challenges

_____

_____

_____

_____

### Questions To Ask & Notes:

## Today's Doctors ♡

## Today's Nurses ♡

## Equipment & Settings:

## Vital Signs ♡

## Medications & Labs ♡

## Feedings & Procedures:

Date: _____

Gestational Age: _____

NICU Day #

## What We Did Today

- Feeding
- Phone Call
- Video Call
- Touch
- Diaper
- Hold
- Skin to Skin
- Check Temp
- Bath
- Visitors
- Photos
- Rocking Chair
- Sing
- Read
- Massage

Today's Positives ♡

Today's Challenges

Questions To Ask & Notes:

## Today's Doctors ♡

## Today's Nurses ♡

## Equipment & Settings:

## Vital Signs ♡

## Medications & Labs ♡

## Feedings & Procedures:

Date: _____

NICU Day #

Gestational Age: _____

# What We Did Today

- Feeding
- Phone Call
- Video Call
- Touch
- Diaper
- Hold
- Skin to Skin
- Check Temp
- Bath
- Visitors
- Photos
- Rocking Chair
- Sing
- Read
- Massage

## Today's Positives

_____

_____

_____

_____

## Today's Challenges

_____

_____

_____

## Questions To Ask & Notes:

## Today's Doctors ♡

## Today's Nurses ♡

## Equipment & Settings:

## Vital Signs ♡

## Medications & Labs ♡

## Feedings & Procedures:

Date: _____

Gestational Age: _____

NICU Day #

## What We Did Today

Feeding     Phone Call     Video Call

Touch     Diaper     Hold

Skin to Skin     Check Temp     Bath

Visitors     Photos     Rocking Chair

Sing     Read     Massage

---

Today's Positives     Today's Challenges

Questions To Ask & Notes:

## Today's Doctors ♡

## Today's Nurses ♡

## Equipment & Settings:

## Vital Signs ♡

## Medications & Labs ♡

## Feedings & Procedures:

Date: _____

**NICU Day #**

Gestational Age: _____

## What We Did Today

Feeding          Phone Call          Video Call

Touch          Diaper          Hold

Skin to Skin          Check Temp          Bath

Visitors          Photos          Rocking Chair

Sing          Read          Massage

---

Today's Positives          ♡          Today's Challenges

Questions To Ask & Notes:

## Today's Doctors ♡

## Today's Nurses ♡

## Equipment & Settings:

## Vital Signs ♡

## Medications & Labs ♡

## Feedings & Procedures:

# Weekly Check-In

## YOUR CHILD IS GROWING IN WAYS
## YOU CAN AND CAN'T SEE

**MILESTONES:**

**UPS & DOWNS:**

**BABY'S LIKES & DISLIKES:**

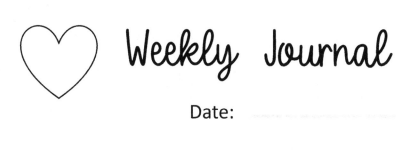

# Weekly Journal

Date:

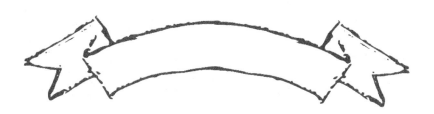

Date: _____

NICU Day #

Gestational Age: _____

## What We Did Today

Feeding        Phone Call        Video Call

Touch        Diaper        Hold

Skin to Skin        Check Temp        Bath

Visitors        Photos        Rocking Chair

Sing        Read        Massage

Today's Positives ♡        Today's Challenges

Questions To Ask & Notes:

## Today's Doctors ♡

## Today's Nurses ♡

## Equipment & Settings:

## Vital Signs ♡

## Medications & Labs ♡

## Feedings & Procedures:

Date: _____

Gestational Age: _____

NICU Day #

## What We Did Today

- Feeding
- Phone Call
- Video Call
- Touch
- Diaper
- Hold
- Skin to Skin
- Check Temp
- Bath
- Visitors
- Photos
- Rocking Chair
- Sing
- Read
- Massage

Today's Positives ♡ | Today's Challenges

Questions To Ask & Notes:

## Today's Doctors ♡

## Today's Nurses ♡

## Equipment & Settings:

## Vital Signs ♡

## Medications & Labs ♡

## Feedings & Procedures:

Date: _____

Gestational Age: _____

NICU Day #

## What We Did Today

- Feeding
- Phone Call
- Video Call
- Touch
- Diaper
- Hold
- Skin to Skin
- Check Temp
- Bath
- Visitors
- Photos
- Rocking Chair
- Sing
- Read
- Massage

Today's Positives ♡

Today's Challenges

Questions To Ask & Notes:

## Today's Doctors ♡

## Today's Nurses ♡

## Equipment & Settings:

## Vital Signs ♡

## Medications & Labs ♡

## Feedings & Procedures:

Date: _____

Gestational Age: _____

**NICU Day #**

## What We Did Today

- Feeding
- Phone Call
- Video Call
- Touch
- Diaper
- Hold
- Skin to Skin
- Check Temp
- Bath
- Visitors
- Photos
- Rocking Chair
- Sing
- Read
- Massage

**Today's Positives**

**Today's Challenges**

**Questions To Ask & Notes:**

## Today's Doctors ♡

## Today's Nurses ♡

## Equipment & Settings:

## Vital Signs ♡

## Medications & Labs ♡

## Feedings & Procedures:

Date: _____

NICU Day #

Gestational Age: _____

## What We Did Today

Feeding    Phone Call    Video Call

Touch    Diaper    Hold

Skin to Skin    Check Temp    Bath

Visitors    Photos    Rocking Chair

Sing    Read    Massage

Today's Positives ♡ | Today's Challenges

Questions To Ask & Notes:

## Today's Doctors ♡

## Today's Nurses ♡

## Equipment & Settings:

## Vital Signs ♡

## Medications & Labs ♡

## Feedings & Procedures:

Date: _____

Gestational Age: _____

NICU Day #

## What We Did Today

- Feeding
- Phone Call
- Video Call
- Touch
- Diaper
- Hold
- Skin to Skin
- Check Temp
- Bath
- Visitors
- Photos
- Rocking Chair
- Sing
- Read
- Massage

## Today's Positives ♡

## Today's Challenges

## Questions To Ask & Notes:

## Today's Doctors ♡

## Today's Nurses ♡

## Equipment & Settings:

## Vital Signs ♡

## Medications & Labs ♡

## Feedings & Procedures:

Date: _____

NICU Day #

Gestational Age: _____

## What We Did Today

Feeding     Phone Call     Video Call

Touch     Diaper     Hold

Skin to Skin     Check Temp     Bath

Visitors     Photos     Rocking Chair

Sing     Read     Massage

### Today's Positives ♡

### Today's Challenges

### Questions To Ask & Notes:

Today's Doctors ♡

Today's Nurses ♡

Equipment & Settings:

Vital Signs ♡

Medications & Labs ♡

Feedings & Procedures:

# Weekly Check-In

## DON'T FORGET THAT THE LOVE YOU HAVE FOR YOUR BABY IS AN INCREDIBLE POWER

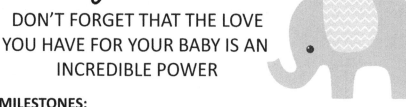

**MILESTONES:**

**UPS & DOWNS:**

**BABY'S LIKES & DISLIKES:**

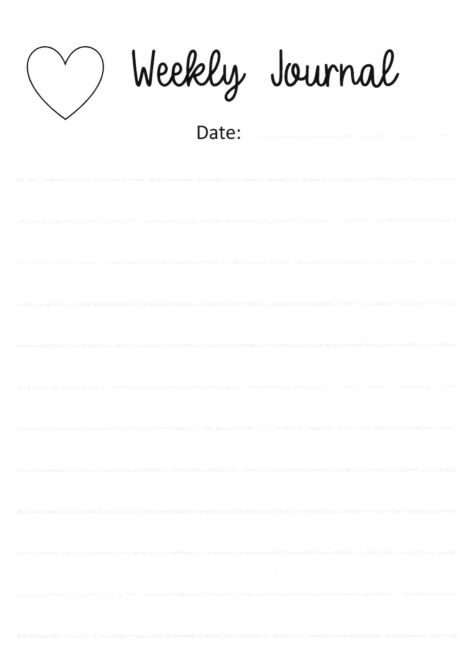

# Weekly Journal

Date:

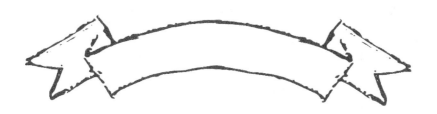

Date: _____

NICU Day #

Gestational Age: _____

## What We Did Today

- Feeding
- Phone Call
- Video Call
- Touch
- Diaper
- Hold
- Skin to Skin
- Check Temp
- Bath
- Visitors
- Photos
- Rocking Chair
- Sing
- Read
- Massage

Today's Positives

Today's Challenges

Questions To Ask & Notes:

Today's Doctors ♡

Today's Nurses ♡

Equipment & Settings:

Vital Signs ♡

Medications & labs ♡

Feedings & Procedures:

Date: _____

NICU Day #

Gestational Age: _____

## What We Did Today

| | | |
|---|---|---|
| Feeding | Phone Call | Video Call |
| Touch | Diaper | Hold |
| Skin to Skin | Check Temp | Bath |
| Visitors | Photos | Rocking Chair |
| Sing | Read | Massage |
| | | |

## Today's Positives ♡

## Today's Challenges

## Questions To Ask & Notes:

## Today's Doctors ♡

## Today's Nurses ♡

## Equipment & Settings:

## Vital Signs ♡

## Medications & Labs ♡

## Feedings & Procedures:

Date: _____

NICU Day #

Gestational Age: _____

## What We Did Today

| | | |
|---|---|---|
| Feeding | Phone Call | Video Call |
| Touch | Diaper | Hold |
| Skin to Skin | Check Temp | Bath |
| Visitors | Photos | Rocking Chair |
| Sing | Read | Massage |
| | | |

### Today's Positives ♡

### Today's Challenges

### Questions To Ask & Notes:

## Today's Doctors ♡

## Today's Nurses ♡

## Equipment & Settings:

## Vital Signs ♡

## Medications & Labs ♡

## Feedings & Procedures:

Date: _____

NICU Day #

Gestational Age: _____

## What We Did Today

Feeding     Phone Call     Video Call

Touch     Diaper     Hold

Skin to Skin     Check Temp     Bath

Visitors     Photos     Rocking Chair

Sing     Read     Massage

Today's Positives ♡ | Today's Challenges

Questions To Ask & Notes:

## Today's Doctors ♡

## Today's Nurses ♡

## Equipment & Settings:

## Vital Signs ♡

## Medications & Labs ♡

## Feedings & Procedures:

Date: _____

Gestational Age: _____

NICU Day #

## What We Did Today

| | | |
|---|---|---|
| Feeding | Phone Call | Video Call |
| Touch | Diaper | Hold |
| Skin to Skin | Check Temp | Bath |
| Visitors | Photos | Rocking Chair |
| Sing | Read | Massage |
| | | |

Today's Positives ♡

Today's Challenges

Questions To Ask & Notes:

## Today's Doctors ♡

## Today's Nurses ♡

## Equipment & Settings:

## Vital Signs ♡

## Medications & Labs ♡

## Feedings & Procedures:

Date: _____

Gestational Age: _____

NICU Day #

## What We Did Today

- Feeding
- Touch
- Skin to Skin
- Visitors
- Sing

- Phone Call
- Diaper
- Check Temp
- Photos
- Read

- Video Call
- Hold
- Bath
- Rocking Chair
- Massage

## Today's Positives

## Today's Challenges

## Questions To Ask & Notes:

## Today's Doctors ♡

## Today's Nurses ♡

## Equipment & Settings:

## Vital Signs ♡

## Medications & Labs ♡

## Feedings & Procedures:

Date: _____

Gestational Age: _____

NICU Day #

## What We Did Today

- [ ] Feeding
- [ ] Phone Call
- [ ] Video Call
- [ ] Touch
- [ ] Diaper
- [ ] Hold
- [ ] Skin to Skin
- [ ] Check Temp
- [ ] Bath
- [ ] Visitors
- [ ] Photos
- [ ] Rocking Chair
- [ ] Sing
- [ ] Read
- [ ] Massage
- [ ] 
- [ ] 
- [ ] 

Today's Positives

Today's Challenges

Questions To Ask & Notes:

## Today's Doctors ♡

## Today's Nurses ♡

## Equipment & Settings:

## Vital Signs ♡

## Medications & Labs ♡

## Feedings & Procedures:

# Weekly Check-In

## BIG JOURNEYS BEGIN WITH SMALL STEPS

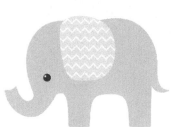

**MILESTONES:**

**UPS & DOWNS:**

**BABY'S LIKES & DISLIKES:**

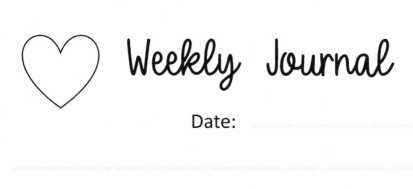

# Weekly Journal

Date:

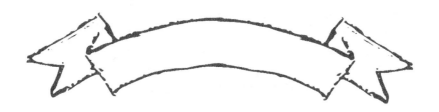

Date: _____

Gestational Age: _____

NICU Day #

## What We Did Today

Feeding         Phone Call         Video Call

Touch           Diaper             Hold

Skin to Skin    Check Temp         Bath

Visitors        Photos             Rocking Chair

Sing            Read               Massage

Today's Positives ♡        Today's Challenges

Questions To Ask & Notes:

## Today's Doctors ♡

## Today's Nurses ♡

## Equipment & Settings:

## Vital Signs ♡

## Medications & Labs ♡

## Feedings & Procedures:

Date: _____

Gestational Age: _____

NICU Day #

## What We Did Today

- Feeding
- Touch
- Skin to Skin
- Visitors
- Sing

- Phone Call
- Diaper
- Check Temp
- Photos
- Read

- Video Call
- Hold
- Bath
- Rocking Chair
- Massage

Today's Positives ♡ | Today's Challenges

Questions To Ask & Notes:

## Today's Doctors ♡

## Today's Nurses ♡

## Equipment & Settings:

## Vital Signs ♡

## Medications & Labs ♡

## Feedings & Procedures:

Date: _____

NICU Day #

Gestational Age: _____

## What We Did Today

- Feeding
- Phone Call
- Video Call
- Touch
- Diaper
- Hold
- Skin to Skin
- Check Temp
- Bath
- Visitors
- Photos
- Rocking Chair
- Sing
- Read
- Massage

## Today's Positives ♡

## Today's Challenges

## Questions To Ask & Notes:

## Today's Doctors ♡

## Today's Nurses ♡

## Equipment & Settings:

## Vital Signs ♡

## Medications & Labs ♡

## Feedings & Procedures:

Date: _____

NICU Day #

Gestational Age: _____

## What We Did Today

Feeding     Phone Call     Video Call

Touch     Diaper     Hold

Skin to Skin     Check Temp     Bath

Visitors     Photos     Rocking Chair

Sing     Read     Massage

Today's Positives ♡     Today's Challenges

Questions To Ask & Notes:

Today's Doctors ♡

Today's Nurses ♡

Equipment & Settings:

Vital Signs ♡

Medications & Labs ♡

Feedings & Procedures:

Date: _____

Gestational Age: _____

NICU Day #

## What We Did Today

- Feeding
- Touch
- Skin to Skin
- Visitors
- Sing

- Phone Call
- Diaper
- Check Temp
- Photos
- Read

- Video Call
- Hold
- Bath
- Rocking Chair
- Massage

Today's Positives ♡

Today's Challenges

Questions To Ask & Notes:

## Today's Doctors ♡

## Today's Nurses ♡

## Equipment & Settings:

## Vital Signs ♡

## Medications & Labs ♡

## Feedings & Procedures:

Date: _____

Gestational Age: _____

NICU Day #

## What We Did Today

| | | |
|---|---|---|
| Feeding | Phone Call | Video Call |
| Touch | Diaper | Hold |
| Skin to Skin | Check Temp | Bath |
| Visitors | Photos | Rocking Chair |
| Sing | Read | Massage |
| | | |

Today's Positives ♡   Today's Challenges

Questions To Ask & Notes:

## Today's Doctors ♡

## Today's Nurses ♡

## Equipment & Settings:

## Vital Signs ♡

## Medications & Labs ♡

## Feedings & Procedures:

Date: _____

NICU Day #

Gestational Age: _____

## What We Did Today

- [ ] Feeding
- [ ] Phone Call
- [ ] Video Call
- [ ] Touch
- [ ] Diaper
- [ ] Hold
- [ ] Skin to Skin
- [ ] Check Temp
- [ ] Bath
- [ ] Visitors
- [ ] Photos
- [ ] Rocking Chair
- [ ] Sing
- [ ] Read
- [ ] Massage

### Today's Positives ♡

### Today's Challenges

### Questions To Ask & Notes:

## Today's Doctors ♡

## Today's Nurses ♡

## Equipment & Settings:

## Vital Signs ♡

## Medications & Labs ♡

## Feedings & Procedures:

# Weekly Check-In

## MIRACLES ARE OFTEN DISGUISED AS PREEMIES

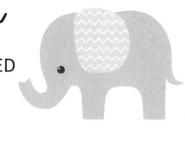

**MILESTONES:**

**UPS & DOWNS:**

**BABY'S LIKES & DISLIKES:**

# Weekly Journal

Date:

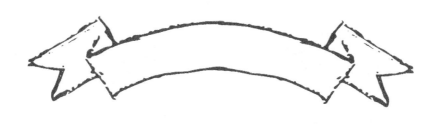

# Homecoming

Date of Discharge: _____

Gestational Age: _____

Time: _____

Weight: _____

Length: _____

Days in NICU: _____

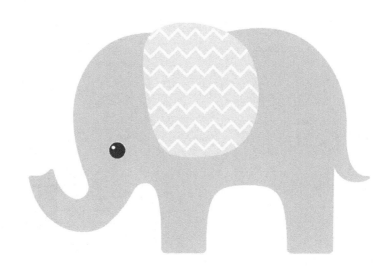

.

Made in the USA
Monee, IL
24 November 2020